9 Day Smoothie Cleansing Diet
Easiest Fastest ways to Lose Weight
By Chris Joseph
Copyright 2014

Who I wrote this book for

When I was doing this *9 day smoothie cleansing diet* I thought to myself this is a cinch I need to get the word out about this. Here it is in this one book. I give you some advice and tips on what to plan for, what to expect and even what products to purchase. I have personally ingested every single ingredient and smoothie in this book and I can say with firsthand knowledge that everything tastes good. If you are ready to lose weight, feel good and look like a million dollars this book is written for you.

This diet is for beginners as well as those of you who may perhaps be "hard losers". The diet itself is a rinse and repeat type of regime. You do the smoothie's the first three days then repeat them for the next days on the *9 day smoothie cleansing diet*. It is very simple and if you follow the directions the amount of weight you can lose is virtually unlimited. Do what it says in this book and you will be on the *fast track* to a brand new you.

I recommend that you be prepared to do the *9 day smoothie cleansing diet*. If you are not ready to make the full commitment to do a diet like this, I encourage you to wait until you are. The prep part of this diet is not fun however you need to get your body cleaned out and prepared to start new again. The prep part of this diet will certainly be doing that for you I assure you.

So if you're ready to put your best foot forward and give yourself a boost in the way your body looks and feels I encourage you to begin as soon as possible. One thing I can say though is that if it is around the holidays and you bought this book or received it as a gift I would tell you to wait until after the holidays are done to begin this *9 day smoothie cleansing diet*.

WARNING: If you have any kind of nut allergies you should omit the peanut butter called for in the recipes in this book. Consuming any kind of nut product can cause an allergic reaction and even death by consuming nuts or nut based products.

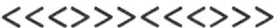

Section 1

Information you should know before you start your diet

You wouldn't consider heading out on vacation without knowing a few things about your travels before you start packing your car. You'd want to know something about available motels, places to eat, and activities that are available. Just like planning a vacation, there is certain information you should know before you start that weight loss diet.

In fact, the reason why so many diets fail is because most people who diet start their diets with only a vague idea of wanting to lose weight without really understanding the exact point they are starting from or what they need to know to successful plan their diet. If you are serious about losing weight here is some information you will need to know before choosing or forming your diet plan.

Know your current daily calorie Intake

By now every dieter knows that in order to lose weight they need to consume fewer calories. But in order to know how many and what types of calories you can safely cut from your daily diet, you first need to know what your current daily calorie intake is, and where you can shave calories without reducing necessary nutrients. So just how do you learn what your daily calorie intake is? Start by keeping a food journal prior to starting your diet.

You're food journal

When keeping a pre-diet food journal, you need to eat the foods you normally do in the same amounts you are used to eating them. Record what you eat and drink for each meal, and all those in between meal snacks. You will need to keep the journal for a week or two to get a good idea of your average calorie intake.

Once you have completed the journal, go through and record the calories you consumed each and every day. Total the overall calorie consumption for the entire period and then divide it by the number of days you kept your journal to get your average DCI.

Once you know what your current DCI (or daily calorie intake) is, then go through your journal again and circle all the junk food like soda pop, chips, candy and cake you consumed each day. (You can average these too.) Then subtract these calories from your DCI and that will give you a good idea of how many less calorie you can consume each day without suffering a loss of nutrients.

If this amount is not enough to meet your weekly weight loss goals, then you could look to see where else you can cut extra calories by eating smaller portion sizes or passing on things like sauces and gravies.

Having some idea in advance how and where you cut calories will help you to plan your diet program so that you can be more successful.

Body Mass Index

Another thing you should know before beginning your diet is your BMI or body mass index. The body mass index tells you how much fat you are carrying on your body based on your height and weight. If your body mass index is 24 or less you are considered to be within healthy guidelines. If your BMI is 30 or above you are considered obese and need to lose some of that body fat in order to remain or get healthy. Knowing your body mass index is important for two reasons. There are plenty of BMI calculators online you can pick the one you find the easiest to use.

First, it gives you a good indication of just how important losing weight may be to your health and gives you a good idea of the actual amount of fat you are carrying.

Second, there are cases where some people have a distorted body image when it comes to their weight and see they themselves as overweight when they are not. In such cases losing weight may actually jeopardize a person's health. The BMI will give you a realistic idea of whether or not losing weight is necessary and just how much weight you actually need to lose to remain healthy.

Activity level

Another thing you should know prior to starting a diet is your current activity level. Most successful weight loss is a combination of diet and exercise. To burn calories you need to increase your activity level, which is hard to do if you don't know what activity level you are starting at. To get some idea of current activity level, calculate the number of hours you spend sleeping, watching television, and sitting either at work at home.

You can also wear a pedometer to track the number of steps you take each day and the number of minutes you spend in actual physical activity such as swimming, jogging, playing sports etc. Be realistic when looking at your activity level because most people feel they are more active than actually are. Spend some time thinking of ways you can increase your activity levels both in small ways and by taking part in exercise programs, or active sports. Knowing exactly how you are going to increase your activity level prior to starting on your diet will help you combine exercise with your diet right from the start.

Health issues that could affect weight loss

Surprisingly too many people, your current health may have an effect on how quickly or successfully you lose weight. Knowing about health issues or medication that are to cause weight gain or slow weight loss before you begin a diet will help you to set reasonable weight loss goals and not get discouraged when you actually start dieting. Before starting any weight loss program it is a good idea to have a complete physical especially if you have any of the following problems or issues:

- Insomnia
- Stress
- Unstable blood sugar
- Digestive issues
- Depression or are on anti-depressants

If you are currently taking medication for any health issues, speak to your doctor and ask him how those medications may affect your ability to lose weight. Your doctor may be able to prescribe other medications or offer advice to help you deal with more effectively with some of these conditions.

Know your food triggers

Everyone overeats from time to time, and most of the causes of overeating can be identified. Knowing your food triggers or what causes you to reach for those salty chips, or that gallon of ice cream prior to starting a diet will help you form a plan to avoid these triggers or at least to effectively deal with them. Food triggers can be any number of things from stress to boredom. Some people's food triggers are certain times of the day or night, others urge to munch or overeat may be simply a smell or a feeling of loneliness. However, unless you take the time to learn what your food triggers are you won't be able to avoid or deal with them when the time comes.

Know that losing weight and keeping it off requires a lifestyle change

Most people think of a diet as short term. However, one of the most important things you need to know and understand prior to beginning a diet is that there is nothing short term about losing weight and keeping it off. To before truly successful with your weight loss requires you to permanently change your lifestyle.

Changing your lifestyle requires real dedication and commitment. It means choosing a weight loss program that is versatile and is customized to your likes, dislikes and your body's needs. It means learning about the nutritional value of foods, and how to prepare them in the healthiest way possible. It also may mean making changes in your exercise routine, your holiday celebrations, and your sleep habits, possibly some of your friends and the entire way you look at food and in some cases life in general.

Changing your lifestyle won't be easy and it won't be something you can do all at once. It will best be accomplished by making little changes getting use to those changes, and then making more changes. It will also take some trial and error to make the necessary changes.

Know that you are not alone

The last thing you need to know before beginning your weight loss journey is the simple fact that you are not alone. Losing weight can often seem lonely and there will times when you feel you that you are the only person struggling with weight issues and no one knows what you are going through. However, there are thousands of people each year who begin diets, and there are support groups both online and off line that can offer you emotional support, advice, or simply a shoulder to cry on. Finding some type of support prior to starting your weight loss program can help to motivate you and keep you motivated.

Finding people who support your efforts and are there when you feel weak can make a huge difference when you are trying to lose weight, and the more weight you have to lose the more important having support becomes.

Now that you have some idea what is important to know before you actually begin that weight loss program, you are ready to start planning for this new adventure and the new improved you!

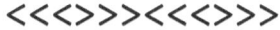

Begin your diet with the end in mind- "The Power of Visualization"

Often times diets fail not because of a lack of commitment or dedication, but simply because the person trying to lose weight simply cannot "see" themselves with a smaller healthier body. For many people learning to begin a diet or weight loss program with the end clearly in mind can dramatically increase the chances of success. How does one begin a diet with the end clearly in mind? Through the power of visualization. When you can actually see the end result in your mind's eye than you can achieve the result you are seeing.

What is visualization?

Used in sports, business and other areas of life visualization is a technique that allows individuals to set the stage for their success and show them what the end result of their efforts can be. For example, a football star may picture in his mind making a winning touchdown over and over again. During the visualization process he can actually picture himself, reaching up catching the ball, running the length of the field and into the end zone. Visualization is a way of creating a pathway in your brain to get the results you want.

For dieters being able to picture yourself with your new body, shopping for clothes, running a marathon or doing other activities that are currently beyond you helps you to actually believe that you can achieve this goal. By visualizing the end result over and over and the steps you will take to get there you create in your mind the belief that what you see is meant to be and believing you will reach your goal is half the weight loss battle.

Believing what could be

If you are overweight, especially if you have been overweight for a long period of time, chances are that you have tried diet after diet without much success. You see yourself as fat or overweight and it is difficult to imagine yourself being any other way. By holding onto this view of yourself, you also hold onto a self-defeating attitude whether you are aware of this attitude or not and therefore set yourself up for failure simply because you cannot shake the belief that this is how you are meant to be.

Through the practice of visualization you begin to change your view of yourself from how you look now to believing how you could look and feel. While it does take practice you begin to slowly picture yourself as a thinner person doing those activities that thinner people do. You begin by picturing yourself at your ideal weight shopping for clothes, going out dancing with friends and enjoying exercising and eating healthy. Keep practicing and until you call to mind this picture of yourself anytime, anywhere.

Mentally watch the pounds melt away

Once you can easily visualize the new and smaller you, then you need to go back and visualize getting from where you are now to that slimmer trimmer version of you. Picture yourself getting up in the morning, stepping on the scales, and seeing those pounds melt away. Envision going through your day happily functioning and joining in various exercise programs and activities. You should even visualize yourself sitting down and eating and stopping the moment you feel sated. Actually picture yourself pushing that half full plate away, or walking past that pastry shop and now feeling any desire to linger, look in the window or step inside.

Visualizing each step you will successfully complete on your weight loss journey will help you to actually succeed at each step. The clearer you can picture each step of your journey to weight loss, the easier it is to take each step in reality. Visualizing helps you build a confidence that you can reach your goal, keeps your mind focused on the job at hand, and paves the way for you to intuitively move in the direction you want to go.

The visualization process

Everyone does at least some visualization whether they are aware of it or not. However, you want to be aware of the visualization process in order to use it as a weight loss weight. Start by finding a comfortable and quiet place to sit or lay down. Close your eyes and breathe slowly and deeply to clear your mind, when you are ready, picture yourself having reached your realistic weight goal. Hold that image in your mind for 10 minutes or more if possible.

- Then start visualizing each step of the process from shopping for healthy foods and preparing it, to sitting down and eating more fruits and vegetables and feeling full and satisfied.
- Picture yourself talking a long walk after dinner, or working out for 20 minutes on that new treadmill and feeling great when you have finished. Actually visualize yourself turning off the television and going to work out. Form a clear picture in your mind of what you are going to do and exactly how you are going to do it.
- Visualize someone offering you a piece a candy or a cake and turning it down and asking for a piece of fruit instead.
- Picture the strategies you will use to overcome temptations and emotional eating, and then picture using those strategies to successfully avoid reaching for those high calorie snacks. For example, if you feel the urge to snack when you feel tense, start picturing yourself going for a walk around the block, or taking a hot shower instead, Feel yourself relax and the urge to eat disappear.

Once you start making healthier choices in your mind, your actions are more likely to follow your thoughts and visions.

Positive thoughts lead to positive actions

Studies have shown that mind is unable to tell the difference between what you imagine and what is real and it responds accordingly. For example, when you continually imagine yourself at your ideal weight, your mind believes that you are that weight and you begin to act in accordance with that visual image of yourself. When you find yourself turning down that piece of cake because you are full and it lacks appeal for you, you then experience success. This success then serves to build on itself and you find yourself succeeding more and more. The more you succeed the more positive you feel and those positive thoughts and feelings then begin to work like a snowball rolling downhill gathering more positive feelings and success as you go along.

The hard part of visualization

The most difficult part of visualization is beginning. Most overweight people have viewed themselves negatively for so long, that it takes several tries at visualization to begin to see themselves and their bodies in a more positive light. The simple fact is, that it takes some time to create strong enough positive thought and images to drown out or replace those negative thoughts and image you have held onto so long. But don't give up; keep trying to visualize what you want for a few minutes each day or even a couple of times a day.

After a while you will begin to see that more positive image and that image will get stronger each and every day until it becomes a part of who you are. Eventually, those positive images will begin to replace those negative images you have in your mind and from there on out things will rapidly start to turn around.

Getting help

While some people have little difficulty mastering visualization on their own, others have a more difficult time. If you struggle to be able to visualize your weight loss, then there is help available. There are experts who hold visualization classes as well as CD and other tools designed to help you learn how to productively visualize. It's worth the effort to get the help you need, and learning how to visualize your weight loss will also allow you to achieve other goals through visualization.

If you are not sure how to contact someone who offers visualization classes talk to your medical professional they may know of someone who offers classes or even one on one instruction.

It still takes work on your part

You do need to keep in mind that while visualization can help you to be successfully at achieving your weight loss goals, getting to that ideal weight still take some work and effort on your part. Just like that athlete still practices catching the ball and running in order to make that touchdown he visualizes a reality, you will still have to work on your eating habits and exercise in order to turn that vision of a smaller you into a reality. So make sure that you don't just visualize the end goal, but also visualize how to reach that goal and then take the necessary steps to make that vision a reality. The best way to make visualization work for you is to

- Set a goal and imagine reaching that goal
- Make a plan of how you are going to reach each step towards your goal and visualize actually succeeding at each step.
- Think of the problems or obstacles you may face on your way to goal and picture exactly how you are going to overcome each obstacle.
- Follow through on each and every picture in your mind.

Before you know it you will see those pounds start to disappear.

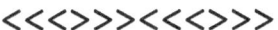

Living healthy is a commitment...Are you ready to commit?

Everything you do in life takes a commitment. Working a job, maintaining a relationship, going to school, all takes a commitment on your part. Living healthy takes a commitment as well. In fact, it takes a large commitment on your part and that commitment needs to be renewed every day. Here are some tips that can help you make that commitment to living a healthier life.

Define what living healthy means to you

Before you can actually commit to living healthier, you first need to be able to define to yourself what living healthy means to you. Do you want to lose weight and keep it off? Do you want to become fitter and increase your stamina and improve energy levels? Do you want to change your complete lifestyle to encompass more healthy habits in terms of eating, drinking, sleeping and other activities? You can't commit to something that you don't have a clear idea of just what you are committing too.

Explore your reasons for your wanting to make the commitment to get healthy

There are right reasons and wrong reasons why people decide to make major lifestyle changes. Some right reasons may be that you want to improve your health and live longer, that there are things you want to do that you currently are unable to do due to your health. A wrong reason might be because your husband or parent is nagging you to lose weight or because everyone else is doing it. Unless your reason for making this commitment is because you want to and you are mentally and emotionally set to make the commitment, you simply will find it difficult to follow through on such a long term and permanent commitment. If you want to live healthier for the right reasons then you will do well to take the following steps.

Educate yourself

Just like you need to develop the right skills for the career you want to commit too, so too you need to educate and give yourself the tools and skills you need to be able to commit to a healthier life. For example is your planning to change your eating habits to lose weight or just become healthier in general then you need to learn something about nutrition, portion sizes and even assemble recipes for healthy meals and snacks. The more effort you put into gaining the skills and tools you need the more ready you will be to make the commitment to living healthy.

Make a plan

To help you prepare to commit to living healthier make a plan on just what steps you are going to take to achieve your goal. Write down your plan and consider each step you will take. Start with a general plan or list. You list may look something like this:

- Eat more healthy foods and eliminate unhealthy foods
- Exercise regularly
- Get more sleep
- Reduce Stress
- Spend more time in healthy pursuits

Once you have a general list of a plan on how to get healthier then take each item on your list one and time and detail exactly how you are you are going to achieve that item. For example take the first thing on your list such as eat more healthy foods and eliminate unhealthy foods and begin to detail how you are going to achieve that goal. Your healthy eating plan might look something like this:

- Incorporate more fruits and vegetables into my diet: Eat at least 4 helpings of vegetables and 3 helpings of fruits each day.
- Include one leafy green vegetable at least once a day
- Drink at least 6 glasses of water a day
- 6 days a week choose lean meats such as chicken, turkey, or fish and one day week allow yourself beef or pork.
- Limit your meat portions to 3 to 4 ounces

- Avoid all processed foods and choose to make fresh meals daily
- Eat a bowl of plain meat or vegetable broth or a single apple before lunch and dinner to cut calories.
- Limit your calories to 1400 per day (or any number that you can set to maintain or lose weight)
- Limit sweets to once or twice a week.

Of course you will want to add more to your eating plan to make it as detailed as possible. While making a plan that details each item on your list will take time it is worth it because it is easier to commit long term to something if you have a clear understanding of exactly what it is you are committing too.

Make preparations ahead of time

In order to help yourself get ready to commit to making the changes you need to make in order to live healthier you need to prepare in advance of making a commitment. If you are changing your eating habits, then throw away that unhealthy food, find healthy recipes to make, and go shopping for those healthier foods. If getting more exercise is part of your plan, then become a member of gym, find an exercise class, or purchase a good sturdy pair of walking shoes.

If eliminating stress then talk to your doctor about different ways to reduce stress, Buy a relaxing CD, or your favorite bubble bath or take a mindfulness class.

Preparing in advance to make a commitment helps you follow through with the commitment you make.

Mentally prepare yourself for the change

Once you have everything set to make the commitment to changing your lifestyle then the next step in the commitment process is to mentally prepare yourself for the change in lifestyle. Being able to view these changes as positive will help set the right tone for committing yourself for the long haul. Visualizing actually having made the changes and imagining the positive effects it will have on your life will help you stay motivated and set the stage for success.

It also helps if you are capable of picturing the obstacles that may arise and then imaging exactly how you will overcome each and every one of these obstacles. By visualizing yourself overcoming the obstacles before they actually come up you mentally prepare yourself to surmount those obstacles when they do arise.

Commitment is ongoing

Keep in mind that your commitment is ongoing. You don't just commit to a healthier life once; it is a commitment you will need to remake each and every day for the rest of life. Just like you recommit to your job each day by getting up in the morning and getting dressed, arriving at work on time, and performing your assigned duties to the best of your abilities, and you must show the same dedication in recommitting to living that healthy lifestyle each day. You recommit to living a healthy lifestyle by the choices you make throughout the day. You recommit each time you turn down that sugar doughnut, force yourself to go for that walk when you are tired or choose to go to bed at a set time rather than go out for a late night with friends.

Each time you make a small decision to recommit to a healthier lifestyle you make the decision to live your goal, and it becomes easier and easier to recommit with each decision you make.

There may be times when your commitment falters and you break your plan. Don't become disheartened, simply pick yourself up and recommit to making the changes you need to make. Beating yourself up over a slip won't help you get healthier, but brushing off that mistake and continuing on your road to health will make you both healthier and emotionally stronger.

Avoid the naysayers

Any time you commit yourself to a goal or a lifestyle change there are going to be naysayers who will tell you that you won't be able to stick to your commitment, or will try and tempt you away from that commitment. Avoid these naysayers as often as possible because their main goal is to prevent you from achieving your goal. This may mean having to drop friends or seeing family members less often, but when it comes to your health you need to stay the course and don't need to surround yourself with people who are determined to keep you from living that healthy lifestyle.

Seek out those who support your commitment

One of the best ways to stay true to the commitment you have made is by seeking out and surrounding yourself with people who are going to support your commitment. Your doctor, nutritionist, exercise buddies, weight loss clubs and groups can all help you to stay strong in your commitment and help to keep you on track. Just knowing that you are not alone and that there are others who have made the same commitment and are working towards their goals will help you to be even more positive about your chances for success. So use these people to help you stand firm and fuel your motivation.

Living a healthy life is definitely a commitment. Are you now ready to commit yourself to making the necessary changes?

You must develop a healthy mindset to diet successfully

Many people decide to embark on a diet because they have a poor body image that makes them unhappy with themselves and their lives. Most people begin dieting with a negative mindset, which sets them up for failure. In order to diet successfully you must develop a healthy mindset. While developing a healthy mindset can be difficult it can be accomplished and here are some tips that might prove helpful in creating the positive mindset you need.

Forget past failures

Many people who decide to diet have tried dieting in the past with little success. These past failures weigh on their mind and they subconsciously think that this new diet will also be doomed to failure. In order to get into a healthier mindset for a new diet you need to forget about those past failures and instead focus on what you learned from those past diets. By thinking of those past diets as a learning experience and focusing on the valuable lessons you learned you can begin creating a positive mindset and a can do attitude that will help you to be more successful at your current diet.

Deal with the issues that you caused or contributed to your excessive weight

For most people there is either a physical or mental issue that caused or contributed to your becoming overweight in the first place. Such issues may include:

- Hormonal imbalances (including menopause)
- Certain health conditions or medications
- Family problems
- Feelings of low self-esteem or loneliness

In order to develop a healthy mindset you need to understand and deal with those issues that caused or contributed to your excess weight. Seeking professional help for any medical or emotional issues may be necessary to help clear up an issue or you may simply have to acknowledge that the issue exists and develop a way to overcome the problems it has created for you.

Develop realistic goals

A healthy mindset includes the ability to set realistic goals for your weight loss. Many people go on a diet after being inspired by those weight loss shows that show people losing an extremely large amount of weight in a very short period of time. However, dieters in the real world need to keep in mind life seldom affords a person with enough spare time to work out 4 hours each day and most people can't afford to have a personal trainer at their beck and call. This means, that you need to truly consider what doable weight loss goals will be for you after considering your lifestyle, your schedule, and any medical issues you may have that may limit your ability to cut calories or the type of exercise you will be able to do.

If you set lofty weight loss goals that will be difficult if not impossible to meet, you will quickly get discouraged and see your efforts to shed those unwanted pounds as a failure. However, if you set more realistic goals that you are capable of reaching, you will start to see some success from the very beginning and this will help to motivate you to further weight loss. My philosophy is now and always has been start small and build on success.

Drop the word diet from your vocabulary

If you really want to develop a healthy mindset towards losing weight then you need to drop the word diet from your vocabulary. The word diet has, for most people a negative connotation attached to it, and using this word has a negative effect on your thinking. Most people associate the word diet with:

- **A short term activity**. When in actually losing weight and keeping it off is a lifelong commitment.
- **Deprivation.** The word diet for most people conjures up images of doing without, suffering from hunger pangs and giving up those foods you really love.
- **Martyrdom.** The word diet is often associated in most people's minds with suffering for a greater good. This leads to self-pity which in turn creates feelings that can cause you to sabotage your weight loss efforts.

Instead, of focusing on the "diet" part of losing weight, focus on the benefits of getting healthier. When you view your weight loss as part of living a healthy life you remove some of the pressure and almost all the negativity from your weight loss efforts. By viewing these efforts as a positive thing that you are doing for yourself, you remove the negativity that most people who attempt to lose weight associate with the word diet.

Turn your weight loss into an exciting journey or adventure

Embarking on a new stage of life should be an exciting prospect and something you look forward to not something you look with dread to. By turning your weight loss into an exciting journey or adventure you create the kind of positive mindset that you need to accomplish your goal. There are many different ways to turn your weight loss into something positive and exciting. Here are a few simple suggestions that may start you down the right path.

- If you like to cook, then start looking for those new low calorie recipes that taste good and are fun to prepare. People who do this tend to cut more calories and actually enjoy eating more, as they can use their creativity to create healthy meals that the entire family and all of their friends love.
- Take up a new hobby. Hobbies are a great way to stimulate your mind and crush boredom while getting your thoughts away from food and onto something you can thoroughly enjoy without feeling guilty. Best of all, your hobby doesn't have to be weight loss related as you can join a pottery making class, Take up bird watching, or try that art class you have been longing to try.
- Make new friends. Even if you choose to focus on weight loss related activities such as exercising more or taking nutrition classes, you can focus on the prospect of meeting new people and making new friends who share your interest and your goals and will help keep you motivated.

By turning your weight loss into an exciting adventure you will find yourself focusing more on the enjoyable parts of your journey rather than the challenges which will definitely keep you in a more positive frame of mind.

Don't let the scales define your success or failure

While stepping on the scales each morning can help you stay motivated and moving forward, you should never let the scales define your success or failure. In some cases, especially with people who incorporate exercise as part of their weight loss program there comes a time when you begin building muscle even while burning fat. Muscle weighs more than fat, so muscle gain will result in slowing your weight loss even though you may still be burning a great deal of fat. So keep in mind that the scale is only one tool for you to use. Try to incorporate other tools when determining the success of your weight loss program such as how your clothes fit, or the reduction of inches around your waist, hips, arms, and legs or how loose your clothes are fitting, and how much easier it is to climb stairs, walk a long distance or even jog.

Celebrate your victories

Sometimes when trying to lose weight, especially a good deal of weight people tend to be so focused on reaching the final goal that they fail to celebrate or acknowledge all those little victories they have along the way. Celebrating those victories is extremely important to keeping a positive mindset. Take the time out to acknowledge and celebrate all those small goals you achieve along the way. For example when you shed those first ten pounds why not reward yourself with a movie or having your nails done or best of all a nice relaxing message.

When you celebrate your victories by doing something positive for yourself it makes you feel more attractive and more deserving of those good things in life and there is nothing more emotionally or mentally positive than feeling good about yourself and what you accomplish.

Build upon your successes

It can be quite difficult to maintain a healthy mindset over a long period of time. However, if you learn to build upon your successes you will soon find that it is much easier to stay positive as time goes by. The very fact that you are able to accomplish one goal gives you the confidence to tackle the next goal and as those successes begin to stack up your confidence and your positive mindset will only continue to grow.

Building on your successes also makes it easier to pick yourself up when you experience one of the inevitable occasions when you back slide or splurge on your diet, because you will be able to see these events for what they truly are, a minor glitch in your way to your goal. Being able to view those glitches realistically instead of viewing them as a sign you are destined to failure will make a huge difference in your being able to successfully shed those pounds.

So if you are ready begin that weight loss journey, make sure that you spend some time developing a healthy mindset that will lead you to success.

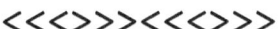

Things to consider before starting any diet or weight loss regime

Most people give at least some thought to the career they want where to go for vacation, and what type and style of clothes to buy. However, when it comes to starting a diet or weight loss regime it seems like most people give little to consideration before embarking on a diet, which may be one reason why so few weight loss attempts are successful. Just like many other things in life there are things you need to consider before starting any diet or weight loss regime. Here are some of the things you need to consider.

Am I ready to make a change?

No one really likes to be overweight, but many people simply aren't mentally or emotionally ready to make the changes in their lifestyle that a weight loss regime requires. You need to ask yourself if you personally are ready to make a change or if you are considering dieting for some other reason such as pressure by family or friends, or simply because everyone else is doing it. Unless you are really ready to make the change for your own reasons, your weight loss regime is destined to failure.

How will my current physical condition affect my weight loss goals?

While there is little doubt that losing weight will make you healthier overall, you do need to consider your current physical condition and how it may affect your weight loss goals. If you are grossly obese, have back or joint problems, or suffer from certain medical issues the amount and types of exercise you will safely will be able to do will be somewhat limited at least in the beginning.

This means if you are planning on using exercise as part of your weight loss program you to consider the type of amount of exercise you can safely do each day and set your weight loss goals accordingly. If can only stand in one place and you can bend at the knees you can lose weight. There is a link to a video coming up that shows you exactly what to do and how to do it.

Do you have the dedication to stick to a weight loss regime?

There is an old saying that goes "When the going gets tough, the tough get going." When considering a weight loss regime you really need to consider whether you have the dedication to stick to a weight loss diet until you have achieved your goals. If you are the type of person that has difficulty completing anything that takes more than a few minutes then you really need to consider how you are going to muster the dedication and determination to stick to diet for weeks, months, or even a year.

What are my weight loss goals?

One of the main things you need to consider *before* starting any diet or weight loss regime is what your weight loss goals *actually are*. You should not only consider the overall amount of weight you want to lose, but also short terms goals as well. These goals should be realistic and based on good nutrition and exercise not fad diets or meal skipping. You should also set enough short term goals that you can reach in short periods of times so that you can see yourself making progress which help to keep you motivated.

Do you have a healthy long range plan?

Many diet plans are geared for people needing or wanting to lose 25 pounds or less. If you have a significant amount of weight to lose than is going to take some time to achieve then you need to consider whether or not you have a healthy long range plan. A healthy long range plan to start with small changes you can make that will start you off losing weight without feeling as though you are depriving yourself. It should also include "free days" where you can take a brief respite from your diet and eat small amounts of foods you crave or enjoy.

A long range plan should also include ideas of how you are will deal with plateauing, when and how to increase exercise to continue to get positive results and how to make permanent and healthy changes in your diet that you can follow the rest of your life.

What obstacles do I need to overcome?

Every person who starts a weight loss program is faced with many obstacles they will need to overcome in order to successfully lose weight. Before actually beginning a diet or weight loss program you need to consider what obstacles you are likely to face and form a plan of how you will overcome those obstacles. Some of the obstacles you are likely to face include:

- Hunger pangs
- Food cravings
- Being tempted by others
- Holidays
- Eating from boredom or stress

Planning how you will overcome these obstacles will make it easier for you to know what to do when you are actually faced with them once you begin your diet.

Have I acquired all the necessary tools to help my diet be successful?

Another thing you need to consider before starting on that weight loss program or diet is what your tools you will need to be successful. While different people find different tools more beneficial to their success the following tools are often helpful to many people.

- **A good set of scales-** Being able to keep track of your weight loss accurately can help you to stay on target and motivated. Scales that show the loss of as little as 1/10 of pound can be especially helpful to people who are easily discouraged
- **Food scales and measuring cups-** Portion control is very important to most weight loss regimes so having the tools on hand to measure out those portions prior to starting your diet will help get you off on the right track.
- **Calorie/carbohydrate counter-** If you are going to be counting calories or carbohydrates then having a book or some type of counter to keep track of how many calories is in food item is a must.
- **Food journal-** Many dieters find a food journal to be an extremely helpful tool when trying to lose weight. Keeping a food journal helps you to see in black and white just how much food you are consuming throughout each day, and helps you identify when you are most likely to overeat so that you can make adjustments to your diet.
- **Exercise equipment-** If you are planning on incorporating exercise into your weight loss regime then you might want

to consider having some exercise equipment on hand before starting your diet. Even something as simple as a good pair of walking shoes or a bicycle can give you a quick start to your weight loss exercise.

- **Collection of low calorie recipes-** Another tool that is helpful to have prior to starting your diet is a collection of low calorie recipes. Having a collection of different low calorie recipes on hand will help provide you with variety in your diet and prevent you from grabbing that take out fast food simply because you don't know what to cook. Your collection should include fancy dishes for holidays and other special events as well as everyday meals and even quick to make foods for time is limited. Having a few low calorie desserts may help to prevent those cravings for sweets.

Do you have some means of emotional support to help you through the tough times?

Every single person needs some emotional support when making major changes in their life. Following a weight loss regime and losing weight is considered a major change and having emotional support when times get tough can often mean the difference between sticking to your diet and succeeding and going off track and ending up back where you started. If you can spend a little time lining up some emotional support prior to starting your diet, it will be there when you need it. Some great sources of emotional support include:

- Diet groups such as weight watches
- Online diet forums
- Family and Friends
- Exercise buddies or diet buddies

How will you keep off that weight?

If you are about to embark on a diet or weight loss program, chances are your thoughts are focused on losing the weight. However, before you actually start losing the weight you need to consider how you plan on keeping that weight off once you have lost it. Yo-yo dieting is not good for your body or morale so having a plan to keep that weight off once it is gone will keep you feeling good about your weight loss and new body. Having a good maintenance program already mapped out before you lose all that excess weight can help keep you from re-gaining any of the weight you have lost and prevent you from ever having to diet again. So take the time to consider how to keep that weight off you are going to working so hard to lose.

Taking the time to go through these considerations prior to embarking on weight loss regime can help keep you focus once you begin that weight loss program. Your best chance of success is formulating a plan of action that you can follow from start to finish.

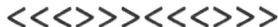

How to physically prepare yourself for your diet

Magazines and even the internet is filled with articles on how to mentally and emotionally prepare yourself to diet successfully, but little is said about the actual physical preparation you can do to increase the chances of your diet's success. Here are a few tips on how to physically prepare yourself for your diet.

Get a complete check up

Before you begin any diet you should visit your doctor and get a thorough check-up. You want to make sure that there are no health issues that could affect your health or your ability to lose weight. You also want to check with your doctor to determine the amount and type of exercise you can safely do. Your doctor can also advise you of any current medication that can affect your ability to lose weight. Making sure you can diet safely before you actually begin a diet, can help you avoid health problems in the future.

Start building up your physical stamina

Exercise is an essential part of any weight loss program, but many people who start a diet simply do not have the physical stamina to exercise enough to burn to calories. When preparing yourself for a diet, you should start taking short walks, lifting light weights and working at other types of mild exercise to begin to build up your stamina so that once you begin your diet, you have the stamina to exercise effectively to help burn those calories and lose weight.

One of the best ways to start building up your stamina is by simply walking. Even if you can only walk five minutes when you first start, if you continue walking each day, you will soon begin to build up some of your stamina and be able to walk further and further and will also be able to engage in other calorie burning exercise.

Clean house/ remove all your junk food

One great way to physically prepare yourself for your diet is to clean all that unhealthy and high calorie food out of your home and replace it with lean meats, fruits, vegetables and whole grains. By physically removing junk food from your home you are also mentally preparing yourself for the beginning of your diet. There is actually something cathartic about throwing away all that junk and fattening food, giving you the feeling of purging your home of unhealthy foods.

In addition, re-stocking your home with healthy food it allows you to visually see the changes you are making, which for many people increases their confidence in their ability to be successful.

Try out low calorie recipes

You can also physically prepare yourself for your diet by collecting and trying out low calorie recipes in advance of your diet. By testing recipes you can find those recipes you truly enjoy and that will satisfy your taste buds and your hunger. It also makes it easier to stick to a diet when you truly enjoy the food that you are allowed to eat on the diet. Having a large variety of tested recipes prepared in advance will make it easier to stick to your diet once you start.

If you experiment with cooking a low calorie recipe a few times a week prior for several weeks prior to starting your diet not only will you have several recipes on hand you really like, you also will be preparing your palate for new foods.

Keep a pre-diet food journal

Two or three weeks before you plan to start your diet keep a food journal. Eat what you normally would, but write down everything you eat in the course of each day. By keeping a food journal, you can easily see where you can immediately cut back on calories to start losing weight. A food journal also allows you to see just how much you are consuming each day, which is important because most people eat far more than they realize.

Clean out your clothes closet

Before starting your diet, you should also clean out your clothes closet removing all those "fat clothes" (clothes you are keeping in case you gain more weight.) By removing the option of something to wear if your diet fails and you gain more weight; you are mentally preparing yourself to not gain weight. The first step in dieting is to prevent further weight gain and getting rid of those larger size clothes will help you to not gain weight.

Purchase an outfit or suit you love in the next size smaller

Another way to prepare for your diet is to go shopping and choose an outfit you really love in a size or two smaller than you are now wearing. Hang that outfit in the front of the closet where you will see each time you get dressed so that it will serve as motivation to stick to the diet so that you can fit into the outfit. Once you start your diet and are losing weight you can help keep your motivation strong by continuing to purchase outfits one at time in a smaller size.

Go on a sugar detox

To physically help prepare you for weight loss without those sugar cravings that are so difficult resist, go on a sugar detox prior to starting your formal diet. You should begin your detox at least 21 days prior to dieting by eliminating all soda's, fruit drinks, desserts, processed foods, candy, and condiments, from your diet.

A sugar detox not only helps your prepare your body for changes in eating habits, it also may have the added benefit of resulting in your shedding a few pounds before actually begin your diet plan. Since the average person consumes about 150 pounds of sugar per year, a sugar detox is a great way to prepare for dieting as your body will adjust to not being fed sugar prior to the start of your diet, which will result in one less issue you will need to deal with while struggling to shed those pounds.

Increase your water intake

Another thing you can do to physically prepare you for dieting is too increase you water intake a few days or a week before you actually begin to cut those calories. Many times we reach for food, when we are slightly dehydrated and really crave water. Getting in the habit of increasing your water intake will help you remain hydrated, can slow your desire for snacks, and will aid in removing toxins and burned fat from your body.

Adjust your sleep habits

Studies show that people who don't get at least 8 hours sleep per night have a tendency to do more late night snacking and be overweight. So it is a good idea to begin adjusting your sleep habits to be more conducive to getting 8 hours sleep a night. By getting in the habit of getting a good sleep you can set the stage to avoid those late night snacks that can sabotage your diet. Being rested will also help to reduce stress which also plays a role in a tendency to overeat.

Develop a meal time routine

While planning your weight loss program starting getting into a set routine for your meals. This routine should include:

- Eating at set times throughout the day
- Learning to sit down to eat your meal and eating slowly savoring every bite. Chew each bit well before swallowing.
- Filling your plate in the kitchen instead of bringing serving bowls to the table. (When food is sitting within easy reach it is easy to reach for seconds without even thinking.)
- Turn off the television, radio, music, and other distractions when you eat. NO PHONE IN YOUR HAND!
- Avoid snacking while watching television or when on the computer. Instead eat your snacks sitting at the table with no distractions. (this helps to eliminate mindless eating)

By developing a good meal time routine before you begin your diet, you start to pay more attention to what and how much you eat. Some people even feel far more satisfied when they eat slowly and savor each bite than they do when gulp down their food or simply stuff their faces mindlessly.

The whole idea of physically preparing yourself for your diet is to begin giving yourself routines and tools and that will make dieting easier once you begin in earnest. By starting to develop good eating and sleep habits prior to starting your diet, you will begin to slowly ease yourself into diet mode, and the changing of your lifestyle instead of trying to change everything at once. Even if it takes weeks or even two or three months to establish and change some of your lifestyle habits before actually starting a diet, that time will be well spent because it will reduce some of the stress dieting can cause.

By physically preparing yourself for your diet you are stacking the odds for success in your favor. The more mentally and physically you are prepared when you begin your diet the more likely you are to follow through and get the results you need and desire.

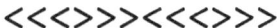

Importance of water in dieting

We all know that every plant, animal, and human needs water to survive. But did you know the important role water plays in dieting? That's right while the simple act of drinking water won't in and of itself result in major weight loss, it is no less an important part of any weight loss program and has many benefits to those who are struggling to lose weight. Here is just some of the important ways water can help you shed those pounds.

Prevents dehydration and helps to reduce hunger pangs

When your body needs to be hydrated it lets your brain know in much the same way as it signals your brain you need to consume nutrients and calories by sending hunger signals. In fact, studies have shown that normal people often mistake thirst for hunger and reach for snacks instead of the kitchen tap. By drinking enough water to prevent dehydration, you can actually naturally cut some of the excess and unnecessary calories from your diet while at the same time preventing some of those thirst signals that manifest themselves as hunger pangs.

In addition, when your body becomes dehydrated, your metabolism and your ability to burn fat slow down. So by drinking water, you can actually keep burning that extra fat more efficiently than you can when you are dehydrated.

Aids in the transportation of essential nutrients

Many times when a person feels hungry it isn't really food that body needs for specific nutrients that may be missing from their diet. This is one of the reasons why diet experts suggest that all people just not those trying to lose weight, eat a wide variety of healthy foods so that they take in all the various nutrients their body needs to properly function. Drinking water aids digestion, which is the breaking down of nutrients for your body's use, and the transportation of those nutrients to various parts of your body. The transportation of nutrients throughout the body helps you to keep you feeling hungry and keeps you healthy while you are losing weight.

Helps to control calorie intake

As you know the key to weight is to take in fewer calories than you burn in a day. Water can help you to better control your calorie intake which results in your consuming fewer calories each day resulting in more and faster weight loss.

Studies have shown that people who drink 16 ounces of water ½ hour prior to eating tend to eat less than those who do not drink water. Other studies suggest that if you eat slowly and drink water while you are eating, the food tends to expand in your stomach resulting in your feeling full faster. In both cases the water, which is completely calorie free, helps to fill you up reducing the amount of calories you consume at each meal.

How many extra pounds can you lose by consuming water before or during meals? No one can really say for sure as different studies have exhibited different results. But even if drinking water only results in an addition 2 or 3 pounds of weight loss over the course of 2 or 3 months, it is well worth the effort, because as every dieter knows, every single pound lost counts and brings you closer and closer to your goal.

Occupies the hands and mouth

For people who are boredom eaters, breaking the habit can be difficult. Whenever they have little to do and their hands and mouth are free they end up mindless stuffing their face. Keeping a glass or bottle of water on hand can give boredom eaters something to occupy their hands and mouth and prevent them from stuffing themselves with chips, pretzels, and other unhealthy snacks. Carrying a glass or bottle of water around at holiday parties or a family get together where is there is a lot of food, especially unhealthy snacks can also help keep your hands occupied and prevent you from reaching for those snacks while mingling and chatting. If you have to set down a bottle or glass of water to pick up food, it gives you that extra moment to think about whether or not you really want that food that you are about to take.

Energizes you and your muscles

People who become dehydrated often feel tired and weak and lack the energy to make it through the day much less take part in exercise programs that will them to burn off those calories. Drinking sufficient amounts of water each day will help you feel stronger and give you more energy so that you can exercise and thus help burn off some of that excess fat.

In addition, water also energizes your muscles which help you to be able to work out longer and with more intensity without feeling muscle pain or stiffness. This enables you to burn even more calories during each exercise session helping you burn that fat even faster.

Helps prevent constipation

Making changes in your diet, even to a healthier diet, can wreak havoc with your body, especially near the beginning of your diet. One of the most common complaints of people during the first days and weeks of weight loss program is that they experience constipation. Constipation not only makes a person feel bloated, it also tends to make them feel weak and tired. Drinking plenty of water can go a long way in helping to prevent constipation and keep everything moving a long so your feel stronger and less tired, and better able to focus on your weight loss goals.

Helps you save those calories for more filling foods

If you have ever dieted before you have probably heard the advice that you need to eat and not drink your calories. Water can help you accomplish that goal. By replacing those calorie loaded sodas and juices with plain water, you can use more of your allotted calories for real foods like fruits, vegetables, or lean meats and healthy grains. This allows your body to get even more of the nutrients it needs instead of wasting it on empty calories.

How much water should you drink?

Every person is different and their body's needs are different as well so there is really no set amount of water that is right for anyone. The rule of thumb for most people (not for those with conditions like congestive heart failure) is to try to drink a minimum of 8-10 ounce glasses a day. However, if the weather is hot, or you are doing a lot of exercise you may need more water to stay fully hydrated. So learn to pay attention to your body's signals and drink water whenever you need to stay hydrated and healthy.

Ways to use water to help your weight loss goals

There are a variety of ways you can incorporate water into you weight loss plan and allow it to help you to reach your weight loss goals. Here are some simple ways of incorporating more water into your diet.

- Drink a glass of water with breakfast. Add some juice from a fresh orange or lemon to water to add a bit of taste and wake you up in the morning.
- Keep a bottle of water with you when walking or doing other exercise and use it to stay hydrated while working out.
- Drink a glass of water instead of a soda or fruit juice with your meals. The water will cleanse your palate and your food will taste better.
- When you start to feel hungry and want a snack, drink a glass of water and wait about 15 minutes to see if you still feel hungry. In many cases the water will satisfy you and you won't need to snack.
- When reading, watching television, or spending time on the compute keep a pitcher of ice water nearby. You can add a few orange, lemon or lime slices to the water or even a handful of berries to give your water a more satisfying taste.
- When arriving at a party or social event where drinks and finger foods are being served ask for a glass or bottle of water and sip on that instead of a high calorie mixed drink or reaching for the appetizer tray.

- Drink a full glass of water just prior to going to bed, this will help you to stay more hydrated throughout the night and you might just get a better night's sleep.

Take a swim

Drinking water isn't the only way you can use water to aid you in losing weight. Swimming is great exercise a wonderful way to burn calories while getting a low impact workout. In addition, many places offer water aerobics which is great way to burn even more calories and meet people and make friends who share the same goals as you do.

Not only is water important to maintaining good health, it is also an important tool to help you shed those pounds and remain healthy while doing so.

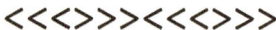

If you can walk you can lose weight and fat

The best way to lose weight is to combine a healthy low calorie eating plan with exercise. However, many people who embark on a weight loss plan seem to find the idea of exercising terrifying and difficult. While you may not feel able to take part in a high intensity workout program, that doesn't mean that you can't make exercise part of your weight loss journey. In fact, if you can walk you lose weight and fat and get in healthy exercise that will build muscle and tone your body.

Walking works for people of all fitness levels

One of the things that make walking an excellent form of exercise for weight loss is that it works for people of all different fitness levels. As long as you can walk, you can burn calories by walking.

While many experts will tell you that you need to walk at a certain speed or a certain distance in order the burn calories, the simple truth is that anytime you move you are burning calories. Of course the longer you exercise and the more intensely you exercise the more calories you will burn, but getting moving even a short distance will help you build up the strength and stamina to exercise more. In addition, studies show that people who walk for their health or for weight loss tend to stick continue to stick their exercise routine better than people who engage in other types of exercise.

No specialized equipment

Walking is also the best exercise for people on a budget because you don't need any type of specialized equipment. All you really need is a comfortable pair of walking shoes and the determination to walk.

Start slow and build up over time

When you first begin exercising, especially if you have not exercised in a long time over exercising can result in sore muscles and a lack of interest in continuing to exercise. So, start by walking at your normal gait for a few minutes. Even walking as little as 5 minutes will burn a few calories and help you to start to building muscle.

Once you can easily walk for 5 minutes or a certain distance you have set for yourself, then start increasing the distance or time you walk. Continue doing this until you can easily walk for 30 to 45 minutes at one time.

Once you are walking a healthy distance, then you can begin increasing the speed at which you walk. As your fitness levels increases you will be able to walk further and faster and may become interested in beginning other types of exercises as well.

You can walk indoors or outdoors

Another good thing about walking to burn calories is that you can walk anywhere or anytime. Not only can you walk outdoors where you can fresh air and enjoy the sights, but you can also walk inside when the weather is poor. There are even DVDs you can purchase that will teach you how to walk in place while burning calories and become more fit.

How many calories can I burn by walking?

When first starting a weight loss routine, you are impatient to burn as many calories and shed as many pounds as possible. So you probably want to know how many calories you can burn by walking. However, the fact is that there are so many variables that go into figuring out the number of calories you can burn by walking. These variables include your current weight, whether you walk carrying weights or using ankle weights, the distance you walk, and the speed you walk that you distance.

A person who weighs 160 pounds will burn 100 calories for every mile they walk. If you walk faster or carry weights you burn more calories, if you weigh 200 pounds you will burn more calories in a mile that that 160 pound person or one who weighs less. If you walk a mile every 15 minutes and walk for 45 minutes once a day you will likely burn 300 calories, or 2100 per week. If you take two 45 minute walks a day you will burn 600 calories or more than a pound a week.

However, you need to remember that your walking will be combined with other calorie burning activities (even sleeping you burn calories) as well as a reduced calorie intake which help you lose more weight than exercise or diet alone. One of my secret tricks to losing weight is to wear a t-shirt a sweat shirt and some sweat pants to bed. Heat burns calories. Try weighing yourself before bed then wear what I just said and then weight yourself when you wake up.

In addition, walking regularly helps to speed up your metabolism so you will be burning more calories faster even at rest. So walking will help you lose weight in more ways than one.

How pedometers can help motivate you to walk

One of the best tools to motivate people to walk more is a pedometer. When a person uses a pedometer to track their steps, they have a tendency to want to take a few more steps each day than they took the day before. This means that when people use a pedometer they actually find themselves walking more and greatly increase the number of the steps they take over time. The further you walk the more calories you burn so pedometers can actually help you to keep burning calories even as your weight drops.

What is the best time to walk?

Another question that many people ask when considering walking for weight loss is what is the best time of the day to walk? The truth is that any time you can find the time to exercise is a good time to walk, but there are some real benefits to starting your day with a brisk walk. Here are just some of those benefits:

- Taking a brisk walk first thing in the morning revs up and metabolism and actually energizes you so that you are more likely to remain active throughout the day. The more active you are the more calories you will burn.
- Walking can actually help curb your appetite so that brisk morning walk may actually have the advantage of helping you eat less throughout the day, further reducing those calories.
- Walking also reduces stress, and stress often slows weight loss and is a main cause of overeating (stress eating) so anything that keeps your stress levels down will be a help when you are trying to lose weight.

In addition, to that morning walk, taking a short brisk walk after lunch or dinner will help your food to digest better and that after dinner walk may just relax you enough to get a good night's sleep. You might also find it beneficial to go for a walk whenever you crave your snack. Not only will taking a walk get you out of the kitchen and away from temptation, it may also curb your appetite so that you won't feel like snacking when you return.

Walking options

Another reason that walking is a good way to lose weight and fat is because you have so many different options when walking. If you are the type of person who enjoys a few minutes of solitude each day then walking gives you the perfect opportunity to spent a few minutes alone enjoying the quiet.

However, walking doesn't have to be a solitary endeavor. You can team up with one or two friends and walk together or join a walking club. Almost every city and quite a few small towns have walking clubs you can join. Such clubs are actually fun to join and the members keep one another motivated. Best of all when you are part of a walking club, you know you will always have someone to walk with.

Ways to get in more walking even on busy days

Probably the best reason that walking helps you to lose weight and fat is because there are ways to get in some walking even on the busiest days when you don't have time to go to gym or partake of other activities. Here are some ways you can use walking to burn off that fat and those calories:

- **Park at the farther corner of the parking lot when you drive to work or drive to the store.** That way you will have to walk to further to get to your office or into the store when shopping and will be burning at least a few extra calories.
- **Take the stairs instead of the elevator.** Not only will climbing those stairs help you to get in more steps but, you will also be burning additional calories by climbing up and down hill.
- **Walk during work breaks.** Instead of sitting in the employee lounge during those 15 minute breaks why not use the opportunity to walk up and down the halls instead. Not only will you burn off more calories, but you will also help to clear your mind so when you go back to work you will feel more refreshed and less tired.

Would you believe me if I told you, that you can even burn off calories and not ever have to leave your home? If you can bend your knees you can lose weight and burn calories every day while you are on this diet by simply doing squats with your own body weight as the resistance. Here is a link to how to do it properly for weight loss: https://www.youtube.com/watch?v=UXJrBgI2RxA I recommend you start off slow with 15 reps and build from there up to 100. Once you reach 100 then begin to do them faster with less rest in between each rep. The faster you go the more calories you will burn. Always maintain your form though and if you start to feel tired take a breather and have some water. I hate working out so this is the thing I choose to do.

Can it be done? Can you do this? If these people can so can you! Check it out:

https://www.youtube.com/watch?v=VPsszzFwru8
https://www.youtube.com/watch?v=8b2JxrsMQpo
https://www.youtube.com/watch?v=2spG-yoVpgs
https://www.youtube.com/watch?v=OgO44jh00iY
https://www.youtube.com/watch?v=hzPzSLjPifM

Regular people like you and me who took control of their life and destiny. It doesn't matter if they did this diet or any other diet or cleanse, the point is that they *DID* it and so can you if you're ready. Are you?

Not only will some exercise and walking help you to burn fat and shed those pounds, it will also tone your muscles so that you will look better in all those new clothes you are going to buy.

What you eat and when you eat- It is important

By now almost everyone knows that in order to successfully lose weight you need to burn more calories than you consume. Most diet experts will tell you that weight loss is a combination of cutting down on the amount of calories you consume and exercising to burn additional calories. However, successful and healthy weight loss is not just a matter of consuming fewer calories. What you eat and when you eat is vitally important to you losing weight safely and remaining healthy.

Making those calories count

Because you will be consuming fewer calories in order to share those unwanted pounds this means that you need to make every calorie you consume count. This means every weight loss program should begin with you eliminating all those empty calories from your diet. Empty calorie foods are those foods that are high in calories and low in nutrients. Foods such as soda pop, including diet sodas, cookies, and candies, sugar, gravies, and sauces and most processed foods fall into this category, because they are high in calories and offer very little in the way of important vitamins and minerals that your body needs to remain healthy.

If empty calories foods make up the largest portion of your diet then you need to replace some of these foods with low calorie nutrient rich foods. Nutrient rich foods include fruits, vegetables, lean meats and some grains. Such foods are not only rich in nutrients, but are also high in fiber for the most part so that you fill full faster while consuming less calories.

Eat a rainbow

When you give your body the proper nutrients it needs to function well, you feel more energized, suffer from fewer bouts of constipation, and don't suffer from those endless hunger pangs even when cutting back on calories. One of the best ways to ensure that you are giving your body all those necessary nutrients is by eating a rainbow when it comes to fruits and vegetables. Your fruit and vegetable intake should include red, orange, yellow white, green, and blue/purple fruits and vegetables. Make sure that include leafy greens among those vegetables, as leafy greens have nutrients that are missing in most other foods.

If you are one of those people who have difficulty making themselves eat vegetables at every meal then try raw juicing. One 8 ounce glass of vegetable juice each morning will give you your entire days' worth of vegetables all in one sitting. But do make sure to vary the vegetables you juice and try to ensure that a least 2 ounce of every glass of juice consists of green juice from kale, broccoli, cabbage, lettuce and other leafy green veggies.

Don't forget those fruits

Fruits are also a very important part of meal planning for those who are trying to lose weight. Not only are fruits loaded with vitamins, minerals, and fiber, but they also help to regulate your system and are strong anti-oxidants that help to keep you healthy and immune system strong. In addition, eating fruit can help alleviate those cravings for sweets, which will help you to stick your weight loss plan. Fruit can also come in handy to help curb appetite. Studies show that eating a medium size apple or pear 15 minutes or ½ an hour before sitting down to meal can result in you're eating less calories, because you feel full. The fiber in this fruit will also help you to keep feeling full longer.

Lean meats

While you should limit the amount of meat you consume at each meal to only 3 or 4 ounces, lean meat is considered by many to be important to healthy diet. Boneless, skinless chicken and turkey breast, venison, and fatty fish like fresh tuna or salmon are all good meat choices. These meats contain a variety of vitamins and minerals, have some fiber and because they take a lot of energy to digest, you actually burn off about 1/3 of calories in each serving just digesting them.

Meat by products

Meat by products such as milk, cheese and butter should be consumed in limited qualities. Cheese, milk and yogurt are healthy in limited amounts but should be low fat with no sugars or salt added. If you are going to have a bit of butter every now and then, make sure you choose unsalted butter because too much salt can harm your weight loss efforts.

Grains

Grains are also helpful to dieters depending on the grain and the amount you consume. Whole grains, unsweetened oatmeal, and brown rice are some good options for those trying to lose weight.

Water

While not actually considered a food, consuming adequate amounts of water throughout the day is essential to keeping you hydrated and helping you lose weight. When your body becomes dehydrated your ability to lose weight slows. In addition, water can help to curb appetite and aids in digestion and the transportation of nutrients.

When you eat is almost as important as what you eat

As strange as it may sound, when you eat is almost as important as what you eat. While you can lose weight regardless of when you eat, eating at certain times and in a certain manner can actually help to speed up weight loss.

3 meals a day or more?

Some experts claim that eating three meals a day is sufficient for weight loss while other experts claim that eating 6 small meals a day helps you to get off weight faster. While the experts may disagree on how often you should eat the one thing that they do agree upon is that you need to eat often enough and the right foods to keep your blood sugar levels balanced in order to lose weight successfully.

Eating a large meal made up mostly of simple sugars or foods that digest easily can cause your blood sugar levels to rise quickly and suddenly dropped leaving you feeling tired and sometimes craving sweets.

However, when you maintain balanced blood sugar levels you are more likely to maintain energy levels and feel less hungry. When you limit your meals to 3 larger meals a day it is more likely that your blood glucose levels will swing wildly unless you make sure that you consume foods that break down more slowly limiting the amount of energy that floods your system at once.

When you eat 6 smaller meals a day, you are better able to control your blood glucose levels because you are consuming smaller amounts of food more often which reduces the chances of those blood sugar levels spiking and crashing.

When choosing to eat 6 small meals a day those meals should consist of foods high in fiber, protein or healthy fats or a combination of any two or all three.

How much you eat and when

Studies also indicate that the speed at which you will shed those excess pounds may have something to do with when you consume the largest portion of your calories. Most experts agree that to lose weight successfully you need to start the day eating breakfast.

Some professionals suggest that you if you begin the day with a cup of unsweetened oatmeal, with fresh fruit in it and small glass of skim milk or vegetable juice you will have more energy and be less likely to feel the urge to snack on those high calorie foods in the afternoon.

This makes perfect sense as your body fasts all night while you sleep and your blood glucose levels fall. Eating breakfast will re-balance your blood sugar levels and give the energy you need to start the day. It has been suggested if you eat within an hour of waking that you will tend to eat less than if you wait two or three hours before your first meal.

Eat your largest meal prior to 3 P.M.

If you are sticking to eating three meals a day, your largest meal should be made up of 40% of the calories you are allowed to consume with 30% each going to each of the other two meals. A study in Spain suggests if you consume your largest meal prior to 3 pm you are likely to lose more weight and lose it faster than eating your largest meal after 3 pm.

When you eat what snacks may affect weight loss

It has also been suggested that while you should always eat healthy low calorie snacks when you eat certain snacks may affect weight loss. Some experts suggest you eat snacks such as boiled eggs, and yogurt during the early part of the day because they will help you maintain energy levels and that if you are going to snack late at night you should choose alkaline foods such as carrot or celery sticks to munch on rather than the more acid containing fruits.

In the end losing weight is the same as it has always been, you need to consume fewer calories that you use each day in order to burn fat and lose weight.

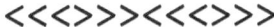

What to eat on "off diet" days. Types of cheat meals that won't hurt your goals

In the good old days, people who began a long term weight loss program were expected to forgo all of those tasty desserts. Salty snacks, and sauces and gravies they loved until they shed every single one of those excess pounds and reached their goal weight. Most dieters found themselves craving those forbidden foods so much, they fell off the diet wagon within the first few weeks or months of dieting. Others managed to reach their goals weight and then went straight for all those forbidden foods piling back on the pounds before the dye and their new wardrobes had set.

Today, diet experts are wiser. They realize that everyone, even the healthiest eater has a craving every now and then for those high calorie, less than healthy foods. They also realize that people on a weight loss program, particularly on a long weight loss program are more able to stick to their diets, reach their goals, and keep that excess weight off if they are allowed to enjoy some of their favorite foods once in a while, under controlled conditions.

Today "Off diet" days or "cheat meals" have become a staple of most weight loss programs, and it actually tends to help dieters stick to their diet plan, and shed those pounds more successfully.

What is an "off diet" day?

First off an off diet day isn't exactly what it sounds like. While these days are meant for you to be able to relax from that stick diet and enjoy a few extras calories and foods you really love, but don't eat on your "on diet" days they are not meant for you to go crazy wild and try to eat every forbidden food on that diet list all in one day. If you are on a 1400 or 1800 hundred calorie a day diet and then on your off diet day cram yourself full of 3500 or 4000 unhealthy calories, chances are you are going to end up feeling sick and too guilty to enjoy those foods you are consuming.

So instead, "off diet" days are designed to help you satisfy a specific food craving, or enjoy a single meal without counting every calorie.

Different people set up their off diet days differently. Some people stick to their normal diet plan and exercise routine during the day and then allow themselves to eat a dinner out, or that consists of their favorite foods. Others simply allow themselves to have a small serving of one or two of the foods they crave the most, while still others raise their calorie limits for the day by 500 or 1000 calories and decide what extras they want that fall within that that raised calorie limit.

How often should you schedule an off diet or cheat day into your diet program

How often you schedule a cheat day into your diet program is going to depend on several factors. Your overall weight loss goals, how fast you want to reach those goals, and the amount of extra calories you will be inclined to consume on these off days. Cheat days like everything else in your diet plan can be adjusted to meet your specific needs, as you go along.

If possible it is best not to schedule a cheat day, until you have become used to your new diet plan and way of eating. For this reason many people don't indulge in their first cheat day until they have followed their weight loss plan for 30 to 60 days.

Most people tend to schedule off diet days once or twice a month and some experts actually encourage their clients to schedule an off diet day once a week. When you have gained enough experience with your dieting you will not even need or want to schedule a cheat day.

What's a cheat meal and what type of foods can you have?

Actually the term cheat day or cheat meal is a rather unfortunate term, since to it conjures to mind doing something that you shouldn't be doing. The whole idea of an "off diet" day is to allow people on a strict weight loss program to enjoy foods they love without feeling guilt, so why use a term that conjures up guilty images? It's better to use the term free meal, or relaxed meal rather than cheat. Regardless of what the meal or snack is called it all means the same thing. You get to enjoy food that is off limits on those on diet days.

While there is no certain type of cheat food or meal that is better than others there are a few rules you would do well to follow when indulging on those cheat days or having a cheat meal.

- **Don't go crazy wild.** It still takes 3500 calories to lose to a single pound and most people only lose between one and two pounds a week, so if you are consuming 3500 extra calories each and every time you have a cheat meal and you have one of these meals every week or even twice a month you are going to slow your weight progress a good a deal.
- **Eat only those foods you really love.** If you have been craving a slice of cheese cake, or some mashed potatoes with gravy don't go off and eat those foods such as chips and pretzels that you don't really miss or want just because you can.
- **Stick to your normal diet most of the day.** Part of the purpose of having a cheat meal or an off diet day, is to help you understand how, once you reach your weight loss goal

you can include these forbidden foods back into your diet and still keep that weight off. Therefore you are still going to want to continue your healthy eating habits most of the day and then simply enjoy a splurge at one meal. You don't want to start your day off with a plate of biscuits and sausage gravy with a side of bacon, have a big Mac for lunch and a large dinner. Instead, you want to choose one of the three meals to add those extra calories to and really enjoy that meal.

- **Stop eating before you're full.** Just because it is an off diet day doesn't mean you have to eat until you are miserable. When eating that special treat or cheat meal, eat slowly and savor each bite, and then stop eating when you feel full. Studies suggest that after the first bite or two of any food our cravings for that food is satisfied, so there is really no need to continue eating that splurge food once your craving is satisfied and your stomach is full.

- **Use diet tricks you have learned to eat less of those cheat foods.** In order to better control the amount of those cheat foods you eat on those off diet days, use some of the diet tricks you have learned to help fill you up before you indulge. Drink a glass of water or eat an apple ½ hour prior to going out for that big meal. Start off the meal with a bowl of clear broth, and skip those bread sticks and go straight for that T-bone and baked potato you have really been longing for.

- **Consider the healthiest way to give in to your cravings**. You should also consider the healthiest way to give into your cravings. For example, if you are really craving something salty you don't have to eat that entire bag chips, or those fatty French fries to satisfy that craving. Instead try sprinkling some sea salt on a tomato or a green apple and you can satisfy that salt craving for far fewer calories.

The benefits of cheat meals and off diet days

There are some real benefits to including off diet days and cheat meals into your diet besides simply helping you to stick to your final goal. These benefits include:

- **A more rounded and realistic diet for life.** While everyone should engage in an overall healthy eating plan. It simply isn't realistic to expect humans to never eat anything that isn't completely healthy for them. We all have food cravings from time to time, and weight loss programs that allow cheat days teach people how to realistically give in to their cravings while still maintaining a healthy diet. It makes maintaining your weight loss much easier when you know have a well-rounded and realistic diet that includes foods of all types, even those food labeled as "junk."
- **Makes dieting less painful.** Cheat days actually makes dieting less painful for many people. No one likes to feel deprived of the good things in life, and cheat days or cheat meals teaches people how to truly enjoy those foods they love, rather than just consuming them.

Establishing healthy eating habits that will last a life time begins with a healthy weight loss diet for many people, and such diets should include allowing for those special treats that we crave in order to help us enjoy a lifetime of healthier eating.

<<<>>><<<>>>

What to do when you have completed your goals - Set more and move on to the next level

When you first embark on a weight loss journey, most of your focus and attention is on one thing, reaching your goal weight. Depending on how many pounds that you need to shed it may take months or even a year for you to reach your goal. There may even be times when that goal seems so far away you wonder if you will ever reach it, but eventually you do. At first, you probably feel a huge sense of accomplishment and pride, however shortly after that burst of excitement you may also feel slightly depressed and find yourself at loose ends wondering "what next? What do I do now that I have reached my goal?"

It isn't unusual for anyone who has focused a long time on a single goal to feel somewhat let down and at a loss when that goal is reached. After all, you have spent weeks and months working hard to achieve success and now that it is here, you simply don't know what to do with yourself. Feeling this way isn't all that unusual especially for someone who has lost a great deal of weight.

Oftentimes, people go on a diet thinking that if they only lost that weight their lives would be somehow be better and more fulfilled. Once the weight is gone, they suddenly realize that their life hasn't miraculously changed, and they end up feeling somewhat let down. The simple fact is that nothing else is going to change in your life unless you are willing to work to change it. The only antidote to that let down feeling once you have reached your goal is simply to set more and move onto the next level. Luckily, for you that are many other things to achieve in life so setting more goals and moving on to the next level shouldn't be too difficult. Here are a few goals you may want to start with:

Maintaining your weight

If you think shedding that weight was difficult, then you may be surprised to discover that maintaining that new weight can be just as difficult unless you have a plan on how you will accomplish that. One way of course is through a maintenance diet that you will need to follow for life. Another way is to find more fun ways to keep incorporating exercise in your diet. Of course with your newer smaller body that are plenty of options open to you. For example you can:

- Take dance lessons to help keep you shape
- Join a walking club
- Train for a ½ marathon
- Take up a sport such as tennis, golf, or even join a softball or baseball club

Share your experiences

You may have succeeded with your weight loss, but there are many people who are still struggling with theirs. Why not set a goal to share your experiences with others and help them to reach their weight loss goals as well. There are many clubs and organizations who try and help people who are struggling with weight, and these organizations often cry out for volunteers. Imagine what it would be like if you shared your own struggle with excess weight with others and could help another person reach their dream as well.

Or why not volunteer to start a after school program for kids who are overweight and start teaching them good habits now so they won't have to struggle later in life. Many schools are trying to deal with childhood obesity and would welcome the help from someone who has real life experience.

There are a variety of ways that you can share your experience with others and doing so will actually help you to understand just how much you really accomplished.

You've improved your body why not improve your mind?

Losing weight is one of the most difficult things that anyone can do. Having accomplished that may just give you the self-esteem and confidence to improve your mind by going back to school, taking special courses, or even seeking a new and better job. One of the things about being human is that is always something about ourselves we could improve and looking for new ways to constantly improve ourselves can keep us motivated and give our life direction. Of course you don't need to engage in formal education to improve your mind, you can join a book club, or other type of club where you can learn how to do something new and meet new people and share ideas.

Set new career goals

You have just finishing spending a lot of time on your weight loss goals and now that you've reached that goal why not set yourself some new career goals to focus on. Studies show that people who really like their job and feel that are doing something worthwhile are far happier than those who feel they are stuck in a dead end job. So why not set your sights on improving your career either climbing up the career ladder where you at now, or looking for a career you would really enjoy.

Setting new goals

Just like you did when considering losing weight, you can set yourself a new goal unless you have some idea what you want to achieve. Spend a little time considering what new goal you want to reach and then start planning how you are going to reach that goal. You will find that many of the lessons you learned on your weight loss journey can be used when trying to attain other goals.

When you select your new goal then start the process of visualizing that goals, identifying the possible obstacles and visualizing how to overcome them, physically, mentally, and emotionally preparing yourself to reach those goals, and gaining the support you need to help keep you motivated and moving forward.

Use what you have learned

The truth is that you learned a lot of valuable lessons through your weight loss journey and you can now use some of those lessons in achieve other goals in your life. These new goals will be easier to reach because you won't be reinventing the wheel; you will be taking those tools you have picked up doing your dieting and applying them to other areas in life. Concentrate on those tools, and figure out how they can help you this new situation to reach new and loftier goals. You have learned so many useful things including:

- The importance of commitment
- How to maintain focus
- How to build on your achievements
- How to put yourself into a positive frame of mind
- How to power through the tough times
- How to find groups or even one person to lend emotional support and the importance of having that support.
- That there are no real short cuts to success.

When you think about it, your weight loss journey has given you all the tools to be successful in anything you endeavor to do in life. All you need to do is to use those tools and you can make any changes you want.

Not everyone needs to have lofty goals

You do need to keep in mind that not all people need to have lofty goals. Sometimes just living a simple life and being happy with oneself is all that is needed. However, even then you will need to set goals to achieve the kind of life and happiness you seek, some of those goals will be short range goals, such as purchasing a new wardrobe to go with your new body, or learning to take better care of your hair or skin.

Other goals will be long range such as raising healthy, happy children, or giving back to society. The most important thing is being able to identify those goals and being able to keep moving forward in order to achieve them.

Don't worry if you can't set a new goal immediately

Don't worry if you can't set a new goal for yourself immediately. Sometimes it pays to take a little time to decide what we want to do next or where we want to go from here. It's all right to enjoy the success you just had for a little while as long as you don't let this one success be the end of your quest. The whole point of successfully losing weight, besides having a smaller body, is learning that you can achieve whatever you set out to do, and having learned that lesson you will soon be eager to tackle new things and to achieve new goals.

So go ahead enjoy your success and when you are ready you will probably come up with many new goals you that you want to achieve and you now know that you have the tools and stamina to achieve those goals.

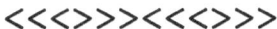

Section 2

Now for the yummy stuff

WARNING: If you have any kind of nut allergies you should omit the peanut butter called for in the recipes in this book. Consuming any kind of nut product can cause an allergic reaction and even death by consuming nuts or nut based products.

Directions for this diet are very simple and straight forward. All you need to do is blend up the smoothies with the ingredients and drink them. You drink water before and directly after you drink the smoothie. The best part about this diet is that that you can do it 3 times in a month and you get 6 days to eat regular food albeit in the proper proportions and the proper foods. I suggest you only weight yourself one time at the beginning of the regime the morning of the first day and the day after you do the castor oil prep. When you have completed the entire *9 day smoothie cleansing diet* weight yourself and journal your results.

I have consumed every single one of these smoothies as they are my own recipes and the ingredients are available at any fruit market or super market in the world. There are some additions that you can make to the smoothies if you like however again most of those ingredients for the additions are available at any health food store or certainly on Amazon.

One thing you can do if you have a busy schedule is to buy 2 insulated thermos containers to take with you to work or where ever your schedule takes you. If there is a refrigerator at your work place you can put the smoothies in the thermos in there for when you are ready to drink them. I suggest you do your shopping for the ingredients on the Saturday before the Monday you will be starting your *9 day smoothie cleansing diet* this way all the ingredients are fresh and you have everything you need so there is no reason to have to "run out" to buy anything else. The less time you have to spend at the food store the less tempted you will be to buy things you don't need for this regime.

Again this diet is very simple to follow and the smoothies are great tasting and very filling. They need to be filling to last you the proper amount of time till it is time to have the next one. Snacks in between are not prohibited although not encouraged either. If you indeed get hungry mid-way through the time between smoothies you could choose to snack on any piece of organic raw fruit or any vegetables of your choice. It's best to stay away from any kind of dipping sauces for the snacks if you are doing fruits and/or veggies.

You can feel free to change the smoothie you drink at what time it is due. Example would be instead of the energizing green smoothie for your breakfast smoothie you could do it for lunch if you have a hectic schedule that day and know for sure you will need the extra energy this smoothie gives to get you through your crazy afternoon.

You can switch them around as needed there are no set rules on which one you drink when as long as you take in all three of them and prepare them the right way. I don't put a lot of rules in here because you will know what is right for *you* once you begin to feel the effects of each different type of smoothie and how it makes you feel at the time of day you are consuming it. If you have any kind of allergies to nuts *you should not do* the chocolate peanut butter smoothie, although you could do the smoothie and just leave the peanut butter out.

OK so here we go on your *9 day smoothie cleansing diet* are you ready to feel like a million dollars? Let's do this!

The day before you are going to start the *9 day smoothie cleansing diet* you will need to do the prep part. It is not fun however I strongly recommend you do it if you want to begin to feel the effects of the diet immediately. I recommend you begin your diet on a Monday so that you may do this first part on the Sunday before.

On Sunday morning when you wake up remove all clothing and weight yourself. Drink 16oz of purified water with some fresh lemon squeezed into it, and it does not have to be cold. Drink the entire 16oz. Next take 2 tablespoons of raw castor oil and then immediately drink another 16oz of water with lemon. A trick I use to take the castor oil is to very carefully place the spoon into my mouth and all the way to the back of the palate as far as possible without inducing your gag reflex. The less you taste of this the better and that is the reason the follow up with the second glass of lemon water. The second glass of water also flushes the castor oil down into the area it needs to get to in order for it to begin doing its work. Another trick you can use is to hold your nose when you take the spoon into your mouth and swallow the oil. What you cannot smell you cannot taste.

Now you just have to wait it out. **_DO NOT_** plan to go _anywhere_ for the entire day while doing this prep part of the diet. You will _absolutely_ need to be by the bathroom at all times. The whole reason for doing this part of the plan is to create a clean colon for you to start with. Depending on your weight it may take 20 minutes to an hour for the castor oil to begin doing its work and once it does you will need to be by the bathroom so as not to have any accidents. Take my advice here don't chance it. _Do not_ start this prep and then say "oh I'll just run to the store". You'll never make it and be really upset with yourself that you did not listen to me here. Ask your pharmacist at any local drug store where the ingestible castor oil is located and they can direct you to it.

The amount of times you will need to evacuate will vary once you have taken the castor oil. Once you start to only evacuate clear fluids only you will be in business. You can follow up in between evacuations with more lemon water as it is soothing to the bowel at this juncture and will aid in the cleansing process as well as keeping you well hydrated. It will be a good part of the day that this will take to complete and you could plan to have some nice homemade chicken soup for dinner if you like but you should not plan to have a heavy meal that includes meats.

WARNING: If you have any kind of nut allergies you should omit the peanut butter called for in the recipes in this book. Consuming any kind of nut product can cause an allergic reaction and even death by consuming nuts or nut based products.

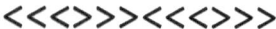

Day 1 on the 9 day smoothie cleansing diet

Prepare your morning smoothie as the directions indicate. Drink the smoothie right away and follow up with 16oz of lemon water immediately.

Directions for day 1 morning smoothie:

Before drinking the smoothie drink 16oz of the lemon water.

Juice 1 bunch of spring mix greens in your juicer along with half of one cucumber, two carrots, two celery stalks, 1 apple, one orange, and one pear. In your blender place 4 bananas 2 tbsp. of raw organic honey, a pinch of your favorite sea salt, 1/8 teaspoon of organic raw vanilla. Place the juice you made in the juicer in the blender and blend on high speed until smooth. Drink the smoothie right away. The produce will be cold from having been stored in the refrigerator so you should not have to add any ice although you can add 2-3 ice cubes if you like it colder. You will have to play with it the first few times to see how you can handle it. After drinking the smoothie drink another 16oz of lemon water.

In between time snack can be an apple, 2 bananas, an orange, or a pear.

Directions for day 1 afternoon lunch smoothie:

Before drinking the smoothie drink 16oz of the lemon water.

In your blender place 5 bananas, 1 cup of frozen pineapple, 1 cup of frozen mango, 1 kiwi, pinch of your favorite sea salt, 1/8 tsp. of vanilla, 2 tbsp. of raw organic honey. Cover with as much unsweetened coconut milk as needed to cover the entire amount that is in the blender. You can also add in 1 heaping tablespoon of flax powder to this smoothie. Blend on high speed until smooth. Drink the smoothie right away. After drinking the smoothie drink another 16oz of lemon water.

Directions for day 1 evening dinner smoothie:

Before drinking the smoothie drink 16oz of the lemon water.

In your blender place 7 bananas, 2 heaping tablespoons of creamy organic peanut butter (if you have any kind of nut allergies DO NOT make or consume this smoothie), 2 tbsp. of raw organic honey, pinch of your favorite sea salt, 1/8 tsp. of organic vanilla, 2 heaping tablespoons of raw organic cacao, 1 heaping tablespoon of regular cocoa powder (FYI Hershey's makes a dark chocolate one now), you can also add a heaping tablespoon of flax powder as you like, pour in enough unsweetened coconut milk to cover. Blend on high until smooth. Drink smoothie right away. After drinking the smoothie drink another 16oz of lemon water.

It is *not recommended* that you have any kind of snack after this evening smoothie. If you feel yourself becoming hungry you can drink 24oz of lemon water.

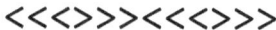

Day 2 on the 9 day smoothie cleansing diet

Directions for day 2 morning smoothie:

Before drinking the smoothie drink 16oz of the lemon water.
Juice 1 bunch of kale in your juicer along with half of one cucumber, two carrots, two celery stalks, 1 apple, one orange, and one pear. In your blender place 4 bananas 2 tbsp. of raw organic honey, a pinch of your favorite sea salt, 1/8 teaspoon of organic raw vanilla. Place the juice you made in the juicer in the blender and blend on high speed until smooth. Drink the smoothie right away. The produce will be cold from having been stored in the refrigerator so you should not have to add any ice although you can add 2-3 ice cubes if you like it colder. After drinking the smoothie drink another 16oz of lemon water.

Directions for day 2 afternoon lunch smoothie:

Before drinking the smoothie drink 16oz of the lemon water.

In your blender place 5 bananas, 1 cup of blueberries, 1 cup of raspberries, 1 cup of strawberries, 1 cup of blackberries, 1 kiwi, 2 tbsp. of raw organic honey, pinch of your favorite sea salt, 1/8 tsp. of organic raw vanilla. You can also add a heaping tbsp. of pomegranate powder to this smoothie or a heaping tbsp. of flax powder or both. Cover with as much unsweetened coconut milk as needed to cover the entire amount that is in the blender. Blend on high until smooth. Drink smoothie right away. After drinking the smoothie drink another 16oz of lemon water.

Directions for day 2 evening dinner smoothie:

Before drinking the smoothie drink 16oz of the lemon water.

Presoak 2 cups of Medjool dates in enough purified water to cover the dates. In your blender place 7 bananas, the 2 cups of soaked dates pitted, the soaking water, 1/8 tsp. of organic raw vanilla, pinch of your favorite sea salt, you can also add a heaping tbsp. of flax powder to this smoothie. Cover with as much unsweetened coconut milk as needed to cover the entire amount that is in the blender. Blend on high until smooth. Drink smoothie right away. After drinking the smoothie drink another 16oz of lemon water.

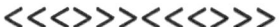

Day 3 on the 9 day smoothie cleansing diet

Directions for day 3 morning smoothie:

Juice 1/4 bunch of kale, 1/2 bunch of spinach, ¼ bunch of spring greens, in your juicer along with half of one cucumber, two carrots, two celery stalks, 1 apple, one orange, and one pear. In your blender place 4 bananas 2 tbsp. of raw organic honey, a pinch of your favorite sea salt, 1/8 teaspoon of organic raw vanilla. Place the juice you made in the juicer in the blender and blend on high speed until smooth. Drink the smoothie right away. The produce will be cold from having been stored in the refrigerator so you should not have to add any ice although you can add 2-3 ice cubes if you like it colder. After drinking the smoothie drink another 16oz of lemon water.

Directions for day 3 afternoon lunch smoothie:

In your blender place 5 bananas, the juice of 5 tangerines, 1 half of a cantaloupe melon cubed medium without the shell, 2 tbsp. of raw organic honey, a pinch of your favorite sea salt, 1/8 teaspoon of organic raw vanilla. Cover with as much unsweetened coconut milk as needed to cover the entire amount that is in the blender. Blend on high until smooth. Drink smoothie right away. After drinking the smoothie drink another 16oz of lemon water.

Directions for day 3 evening dinner smoothie:

Presoak 1 cup of Medjool dates in enough purified water to cover the dates. In your blender place 7 bananas, the 1 cup of soaked dates pitted, 1 heaping tbsp. of organic creamy peanut butter (if you have any kind of nut allergies DO NOT make or consume this smoothie), the soaking water, the juice of 3 juiced apples, 1/8 tsp. of organic raw vanilla, pinch of your favorite sea salt, you can also add a heaping tbsp. of flax powder and a pinch of cinnamon to this smoothie. Cover with as much unsweetened coconut milk as needed to cover the entire amount that is in the blender. Blend on high until smooth. Drink smoothie right away. After drinking the smoothie drink another 16oz of lemon water.

That's it then, now all you have to do is rinse and repeat for days 4-9 with these recipes. I told you this was going to be very simple and it is if you just follow the directions. This type of diet only gets complicated if *you* make it that way. It honestly does not get any simpler than doing it this way.

Your goal can be to lose xxx amount of weight with the first round of the *9 day smoothie cleansing diet*. If your goal is to lose 10 pounds on the first round that could be your goal on rounds 2 and 3 if you decide to do the diet for a whole month. Making your goal each time on the diet for one month would be 30 pounds lost. Do some squats at home then go for a walk around your block and the next thing you know you will look and feel like a million dollars!

That new wardrobe is looking really good right about now isn't it?

<<<>>><<<>>>

Links

http://www.vitacost.com/navitas-naturals-organic-freeze-dried-pomegrante-powder

http://www.vitacost.com/organic-traditions-sprouted-flax-seed-powder-8-oz

http://www.vitacost.com/navitas-naturals-organic-cacao-seed-powder-8-oz-1

http://www.vitacost.com/simply-organic-vanilla-extract-4-fl-oz

http://www.vitacost.com/ys-eco-bee-farms-raw-honey-22-oz-20

http://www.vitacost.com/santa-cruz-organic-peanut-butter-light-roasted-creamy-16-oz

http://www.vitacost.com/funfresh-foods-himalayan-pink-sea-salt-8-75-oz

http://www.walmart.com/ip/Hershey-39-s-Special-Dark-Cocoa-8-Oz/10311958

http://www.walmart.com/ip/So-Delicious-Dairy-Free-Unsweetened-Coconut-Milk-Beverage-32-fl-oz/23591432

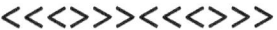

Disclaimer

Before starting any fat loss program, cleansing program or diet you should see a doctor and have a medical examination. The author of this book makes no promises that you can or will lose weight or fat by doing what it says in this book. All information in this book is for educational purposes only and is not to be construed as any type of medical advice or fat loss system.

The author of this book is not responsible for any illness, injury health condition, or any other negative effects which could arise when following the advice in this book. All information in this book is the author's own opinion and should not be taken as fact or medical advice. Acting on the advice in this book should only be done after consulting a physician.

If you have any kind of nut allergies you should omit the peanut butter called for in the recipes in this book. Consuming any kind of nut product can cause an allergic reaction and even death by consuming nuts or nut based products.